ITRAVIL

Begin Your Weight Loss Journey

DR. DAVID FRANKS

TABLE OF CONTENTS

INTRODUCTION

Itravil is a sympathomimetic amine that is mostly used as an appetite suppressant and weight reduction drug. It is also referred to by its generic name, Clobenzorex. This centrally acting stimulant increases the release of dopamine and norepinephrine in the brain and shares chemical similarities with amphetamines. Itravil was created in the 1960s and has been used for many years to treat obesity and associated diseases. The central nervous system is stimulated by the medication as its main mechanism of action, which suppresses hunger and increases energy expenditure. Itravil increases alertness, decreases fatigue, and boosts feelings of satiety by boosting the activity of neurotransmitters including dopamine and norepinephrine. Because of these benefits, it's a desirable choice for people who want to control their weight and change to better behaviors.When managing obesity, Itravil is usually administered as a temporary addition to diet and exercise plans. This medication is recommended for usage in people who have a body mass index (BMI) of 30 kg/m² or above, or in those who have a BMI of 27 kg/m² or higher but concomitant conditions like dyslipidemia, diabetes, or hypertension. It's crucial to remember, though, that Itravil should only be used as a component of a complete weight-loss strategy that also includes behavioral therapy, regular exercise, and dietary changes. Itravil is effective in helping people lose weight, however it is not risk-free. It has the same potential for misuse, dependency, and negative cardiovascular consequences as other sympathomimetic amines. Its use is typically restricted to brief therapy, lasting up to 12 weeks, because of these worries. Overusing it is linked to decreased effectiveness and a higher chance of negative side effects. Itravil use has decreased a little in recent years, in part because more contemporary weight reduction drugs have better safety records. Additionally, because sympathomimetic medications like Itravil can be abused or misused, regulatory bodies have tightened restrictions on their prescription and administration.

Overall, Itravil is still a good option for certain people to manage their weight temporarily, but in order to reduce hazards and maximize results, healthcare providers must closely supervise its use. Like with any drug, patients must be carefully assessed for suitability and given extensive information about how to use it correctly, any possible adverse effects, and the significance of making lifestyle changes for long-term weight management and general health.

PHARMACOLOGICAL PROFILE

Itravil (Clobenzorex) has a pharmacological profile that includes its pharmacokinetics, pharmacodynamics, and mechanism of action. This gives a thorough understanding of how the drug interacts with the body to generate its effects. Because it supports medication development, improves patient safety, and informs clinical practice, this profile is essential for both researchers and healthcare providers.

Pharmacokinetics:

Comprehending the pharmacokinetic properties of Itravil is crucial in order to maximize its therapeutic application and mitigate any potential side effects. The medication is usually taken orally as immediate-release pills or capsules, though there might be different formulations that work better.

Itravil is quickly absorbed from the gastrointestinal tract and goes through a significant first-pass metabolism in the liver after being taken orally. Desmethylclobenzorex is the main metabolite of Itravil, and it has pharmacological activity comparable to the original drug. Due to their significant binding to plasma proteins particularly albumin both Itravil and its metabolites may have different distribution and elimination rates. Hepatic metabolism of Itravil and its metabolites occurs through a number of cytochrome P450 enzymes, including CYP3A4 and CYP2D6. Itravil is transformed by these enzymes into inactive metabolites, which are then mainly eliminated in the urine. Itravil has a short elimination half-life, averaging between 4 and 6 hours, though individual variations may happen. The pharmacokinetics of Itravil can be influenced by variables like age, hepatic function, and concurrent use of other drugs, which can result in differences in drug exposure and response. For certain populations, careful patient monitoring and dose modifications could be required to guarantee the best possible therapeutic results.

Pharmacodynamics:

Itravil's pharmacodynamic effects are mediated by its impact on peripheral physiological processes and different CNS neurotransmitter systems. The main pharmacological effects of the medication are heightened alertness, increased energy expenditure, and hunger control.

Effects on the Central Nervous System:

The main way that Itravil suppresses appetite is by modifying neurotransmitter activity in the hypothalamus, a crucial part of the brain that controls eating habits and energy homeostasis. Itravil stimulates the activation of pro-opiomelanocortin (POMC) neurons and the inhibition of neuropeptide Y (NPY) neurons in the hypothalamus by increasing the release of norepinephrine and dopamine. This results in a decrease in food intake and an increase in satiety. Itravil improves CNS arousal and alertness in addition to its effects on appetite management, which increases wakefulness and decreases weariness. Its effects on the brain's dopaminergic and noradrenergic pathways, which support alertness and cognitive function, underlie these stimulant effects.

Effects on the Periphery:

Itravil has peripheral physiological effects in addition to its central effects, which add to its overall pharmacodynamic profile. These effects could include elevated blood pressure, heart rate, and metabolic rate, along with changes in the metabolism of fats and carbohydrates. Itravil's sympathomimetic effects may stimulate the cardiovascular system, causing tachycardia, hypertension, or arrhythmias in those who are vulnerable. The drug's capacity to activate adrenergic receptors in the heart and blood vessels is assumed to be the cause of these effects, which include vasoconstriction and enhanced cardiac output. Itravil may also have an impact on peripheral metabolism, which includes oxidizing fatty acids to produce energy and releasing stored fat. These metabolic effects, which may be mediated by the drug's effects on adrenergic receptors in skeletal muscle and adipose tissue, contribute to the drug's potential to stimulate weight reduction.

All things considered, Itravil's pharmacodynamics entail a complicated interaction between its central and peripheral actions, which result in decreased hunger, higher energy expenditure, and improved alertness. To reduce the possibility of negative reactions and maximize therapeutic results, these consequences must be carefully weighed.

Clinical Consequences:

Itravil's pharmacological profile has significant clinical ramifications for the way it is used to treat obesity and related disorders. Although clinical trials have shown the medicine to be effective in inducing weight reduction and improving metabolic parameters, there are potential hazards and limits connected with its usage that should be carefully examined. The potential for abuse, dependence, and misuse of Itravil is one of the main issues with its use. It is a sympathomimetic amine, which means that it functions pharmacologically similarly to other stimulant medicines that are frequently misused, such cocaine and amphetamines. Thus, to reduce the chance of diversion and misuse, patient observation and adherence to prescription standards are crucial.

Itravil's cardiovascular side effects, such as elevated blood pressure and heart rate, may also be dangerous for people who already have cardiovascular disease or other cardiovascular risk factors. Before starting Itravil medication, patients with a history of hypertension, coronary artery disease, arrhythmias, or stroke should be thoroughly assessed; in these patients, other weight-loss techniques may be appropriate. Moreover, the transient duration of Itravil medication restricts its efficacy as a sustained approach to managing obesity. Even though the medication may provide noticeable weight loss during the first few months of treatment, its effectiveness usually wanes with time, and stopping therapy frequently leads to weight gain. Itravil is therefore rarely used as a stand-alone treatment for obesity; instead, it is usually used in conjunction with dietary and lifestyle changes.

To sum up, Itravil's pharmacological profile offers significant insights into its pharmacokinetics, pharmacodynamics, and mechanism of action. These insights enhance clinical practice and help guide therapy options for obesity and related diseases. However, in order to minimize dangers and maximize patients' therapeutic success, its use needs to be carefully controlled.

MECHANISM OF ACTION

Itravil (Clobenzorex) works by intricately interacting with the central nervous system's (CNS) neurotransmitter systems, especially those that regulate dopamine and norepinephrine levels. As a sympathomimetic amine, Itravil acts by activating adrenergic and dopaminergic receptors, which is how it works pharmacologically like other stimulant medications like amphetamines.

Adjusting Norepinephrine Levels:

An important neurotransmitter in the body's arousal pathways and stress response is norepinephrine (NE). It acts on adrenergic receptors after being generated in locus coeruleus neurons and released into different parts of the brain and peripheral tissues. NE is essential for the hypothalamic regulation of feeding behavior and energy balance in the setting of appetite regulation. Itravil increases norepinephrine release in the central nervous system by preventing its absorption into presynaptic neurons and encouraging its release from storage vesicles. Increased extracellular levels of NE result from this, and the hypothalamus and other brain areas involved in the control of appetite then experience an activation of adrenergic receptors. Additionally, Itravil's norepinephrine release stimulates the sympathetic nervous system, which has peripheral effects like elevated heart rate, blood pressure, and metabolic rate. These effects are caused by the stimulation of alpha- and beta-adrenergic receptors in the hypothalamus, which in turn modulates the activity of neurons that control feeding behavior, leading to appetite suppression and reduced food intake. These side effects may affect energy expenditure and weight loss in addition to adding to the drug's overall pharmacological profile.

Modulation of Dopamine:

Another significant neurotransmitter that controls motivation, pleasure, and reward is dopamine. It is produced in the ventral tegmental area and substantia nigra neurons, and it is then released into other parts of the brain where it binds to dopamine receptors. Itravil raises dopamine levels in the central nervous system (CNS) by preventing its absorption into presynaptic neurons and encouraging its release from storage vesicles. Dopamine signaling is linked to the brain's reward system, influencing behaviors related to food intake, drug usage, and other enjoyable activities. Increased extracellular dopamine levels result from this, especially in the nucleus accumbens and prefrontal cortex, two areas of the brain linked to motivation and reward. Itravil is known to induce dopamine release, which is thought to contribute to its stimulant effects, which include increased wakefulness, alertness, and cognitive function. Additionally, enhanced dopamine signaling in these brain regions may alter the perception of food reward and reduce the motivation to eat. Dopamine receptor activation in the central nervous system (CNS) raises arousal and improves cognitive function; these effects may be helpful for those trying to control their weight and enhance their general cognitive function.

Other Systems of Neurotransmitters:

Itravil may possibly affect other CNS neurotransmitter systems in addition to norepinephrine and dopamine, though it is unclear how much of an impact these other systems will have. For instance, the medication may affect serotonin release and activity, a neurotransmitter involved in mood and appetite regulation. Itravil may indirectly influence feeding behavior and energy balance by modifying serotonin levels in the brain, though the precise mechanisms underlying these effects are yet unknown. In addition, Itravil's effects on other neurotransmitter systems, like glutamate and gamma-aminobutyric acid (GABA), may also be responsible for its overall pharmacological effects. In the central nervous system, glutamate is the main excitatory neurotransmitter while GABA is the main inhibitory neurotransmitter. Itravil's modulation of glutamatergic and GABAergic neurotransmission may affect neuronal excitability and synaptic activity, which may change how the body regulates appetite and how much energy is expended.

In conclusion, Itravil works by modifying the central nervous system's neurotransmitter systems, specifically by boosting dopamine and norepinephrine transmission. Itravil helps people with obesity lose weight by suppressing appetite, increasing energy expenditure, and improving alertness by increasing the release of these neurotransmitters and inhibiting their reuptake. It's important to remember that the exact mechanisms underlying Itravil's effects on appetite regulation and weight loss are still not fully understood. In order to develop novel anti-obesity medications with enhanced efficacy and safety profiles, additional research is required to clarify the precise molecular and cellular mechanisms at play and to pinpoint potential targets. In addition, the central and peripheral effects of Itravil need to be carefully balanced in order to reduce the likelihood of adverse reactions and maximize therapeutic outcomes. To guarantee the safe and efficient use of Itravil in the treatment of obesity and associated disorders, patient monitoring and adherence to prescription instructions are crucial.

INDICATIONS

The particular medical problems or circumstances for which a medication is advised or given are referred to as indications. Itravil (Clobenzorex) is primarily prescribed as an adjuvant medication and appetite suppressant for the treatment of obesity. Itravil, however, is usually prescribed only to those with a body mass index (BMI) of 30 kg/m² or above, or to people with a BMI of 27 kg/m² or higher who also have concomitant conditions including dyslipidemia, diabetes, or hypertension. Let's examine its indicators in more detail:

Handling Obesity:

Excessive body fat buildup is the hallmark of obesity, a chronic medical condition that can have serious negative implications on one's health and well-being. It is linked to a higher risk of comorbid conditions such as cardiovascular disease, hypertension, type 2 diabetes, and several cancers. In order to manage obesity, a combination of dietary changes, exercise, behavioral therapy, and medication is usually used. In addition to diet and exercise, Itravil can be used to help manage obesity. It is meant for people who may benefit from pharmaceutical therapy to aid in weight reduction and who have not been able to lose enough weight with lifestyle changes alone. As it helps to suppress appetite and reduce food intake, the medication is especially helpful for patients who struggle with excessive hunger and food cravings. The objectives of using Itravil for obesity management are to achieve and maintain clinically meaningful weight loss, improve metabolic parameters, and lower the risk of complications related to obesity. Itravil should be used in conjunction with a complete approach that includes food change, regular physical exercise, and behavioral therapy, rather than as a stand-alone treatment for weight loss, it is crucial to stress.

BMI Standards:

Weight in kilograms divided by height in meters squared is the formula used to determine a person's BMI, which is used to determine whether to start Itravil medication. The use of BMI as a criterion for initiating obesity treatment helps to standardize eligibility criteria and identify individuals who are at increased risk of obesity-related complications. Individuals with a BMI of 30 kg/m² or higher are considered obese, while those with a BMI of 27 kg/m² or higher with comorbidities are classified as overweight and may also be candidates for pharmacological therapy. These guidelines come from organizations like the World Health Organization (WHO) and the National Institutes of Health (NIH). It's crucial to understand that BMI is merely one indicator of adiposity and might not accurately reflect each person's unique variations in body composition and fat distribution. The appropriateness of Itravil treatment is therefore dependent on clinical judgment as well as other parameters such waist circumference, body composition, and metabolic risk factors.

Comorbid Conditions:

Apart from body mass index, the existence of obesity-associated co-morbidities such diabetes, hypertension, dyslipidemia, and obstructive sleep apnea could potentially impact the choice to start Itravil treatment. If addressed, these comorbidities—which are prevalent in obese people—are linked to higher rates of morbidity and mortality. Consequently, managing these comorbidities is crucial for managing obesity and might necessitate a multimodal strategy that includes pharmaceutical therapy. Individuals with comorbidities related to obesity who struggle to lose weight with lifestyle changes alone may benefit most from Itravil. The medication can aid in weight loss and improve metabolic parameters by encouraging appetite suppression and lowering food consumption. This lowers the risk of cardiovascular events, insulin resistance, and other issues related to obesity and its comorbidities.

Therapy Duration:

Itravil therapy is normally limited to a brief period of time, with treatment rounds lasting no more than 12 weeks. This is caused by a number of things, including the possibility of tolerance, dependency, and abuse with sympathomimetic drugs such as Itravil. Since there is little evidence to support Itravil's long-term safety and effectiveness, prolonged use beyond 12 weeks is generally not advised. Instead, Itravil is typically used as a short-term aid to help patients lose weight initially and develop healthier lifestyle habits. Patients are advised to continue with dietary changes, frequent exercise, and behavioral therapy once Itravil prescription is stopped in order to sustain their weight loss and avoid gaining it back. Depending on the needs and preferences of each patient, other weight loss plans or drugs may be taken into consideration for long-term care in certain situations.

Particular Populations:

When using Itravil to treat obesity, several unique populations might need to be given extra consideration. These populations include older adults, women who are pregnant or nursing, children and adolescents, people with specific medical conditions, and people who should not use sympathomimetic medications because of potential effects on growth and development. The safety and efficacy of Itravil in children and adolescents have not been established. Similarly, elderly patients should be constantly watched if Itravil treatment is started since they may be more vulnerable to side effects like cardiovascular events. Women who are pregnant or nursing are generally recommended against using Itravil because of the possible hazards to the developing fetus or newborn. The medication may be excreted in breast milk after crossing the placenta, exposing the infant or growing fetus to the drug's pharmacological effects. Therefore, women who are expecting or nursing should think about using alternative weight loss techniques. In addition, people who have certain medical conditions or contraindications, like heart disease, uncontrolled hypertension, hyperthyroidism, glaucoma, or a history of substance abuse, might not be good candidates for treatment with Itravil. It is imperative to have close contact with a healthcare professional in order to evaluate individual risk factors and establish whether treatment is acceptable for these populations.

In summary, persons with a BMI of 30 kg/m² or above, or those with a BMI of 27 kg/m² or higher with comorbidities, should consider using Itravil for the short-term management of obesity. Its main mode of action is appetite suppression, which lowers caloric intake and promotes weight loss. To achieve the best long-term results, Itravil administration should be combined with behavioral treatment and lifestyle changes. Certain populations, such as youngsters, the elderly, women who are pregnant or nursing, and those with particular medical disorders or contraindications, may require special attention. For Itravil to be used safely and effectively in the therapy of obesity and its related comorbidities, personalized treatment strategies and close monitoring are crucial.

DOSAGE AND ADMINISTRATION

Itravil (Clobenzorex) dosage and administration instructions are crucial for guaranteeing the drug is used safely and effectively in the treatment of obesity. Effective dose strategies, administration guidelines, and monitoring procedures are essential for maximizing therapeutic results while lowering the possibility of side effects and problems. Let's take a closer look at the Itravil dose and administration factors:

Forms of Dosage:

There are several dosage forms of Itravil available, such as immediate-release pills and capsules. The medication is usually taken orally, and dosage recommendations change based on the drug's particular formulation and potency. In order to enhance absorption and avoid gastrointestinal side effects, immediate-release tablets or capsules are meant to be consumed whole with a full glass of water, ideally on an empty stomach.

First Dosage:

When using Itravil to treat obesity, a starting dose of 30 mg once daily is usually advised. This dosage should be taken in the morning before breakfast or as prescribed by a healthcare professional. Depending on the particular patient's response, tolerability, and desired weight loss, the starting dose may be changed. To reduce the possibility of negative effects, dosage modifications should be conducted carefully and under close medical supervision.

Maintenance and Titration:

Following the initiation of Itravil medication, patients should undergo routine monitoring for the advancement of their weight reduction as well as for any side effects or complications. Itravil dosages can be adjusted upward or downward based on clinical response in order to maximize therapeutic effect and minimize side effects. If the starting dose of Itravil is insufficient to produce sufficient weight loss, it may occasionally be increased to 60 mg once daily. Higher doses, however, should be used cautiously because of the higher potential of side effects, such as activation of the central nervous system and cardiovascular events. Itravil's maximum suggested daily dose is normally 60 mg, though certain patient circumstances may call for lower amounts. Once the ideal Itravil dosage has been determined, patients should stick to this regimen for the full course of treatment, which is normally no more than 12 weeks. Extended usage exceeding 12 weeks is usually not advised because of worries regarding tolerance, dependence, and potential for abuse.

Absence of Dose:

Unless it is almost time for the next planned dose, an Itravil missing dose should be taken as soon as possible. In these situations, the regular dosing plan should be continued and the missing dose should be skipped. To make up for a missing dose, patients shouldn't give themselves two doses at a time since this could raise the chance of side effects.

Observation and Evaluation:

Patients should have regular weight reduction progress checks during their Itravil treatment, as well as checks for any changes in vital signs, cardiovascular function, or mental state. Close medical supervision is required to guarantee the medication is used safely and effectively as well as to quickly identify and manage any side effects or complications that may occur. Healthcare providers should also monitor patients for changes in dietary habits, physical activity levels, and general well-being in addition to keeping an eye on weight loss and side effects. In order to help patients adopt healthier lifestyle habits and sustain long-term weight loss success, behavioral counseling and support may be helpful. Regular follow-up appointments are crucial to monitor patient progress, make necessary treatment adjustments, and address any issues or queries that may come up. To maximize treatment results and encourage patient adherence to therapy, open communication between patients and healthcare providers is essential.

In conclusion, specific patient characteristics such as weight loss objectives, medical history, and comorbidities must be carefully taken into account when determining the dosage and mode of administration of Itravil for the management of obesity. Adequate dosing techniques, titration procedures, and monitoring guidelines are required to guarantee the medication's safe and efficient use while reducing the possibility of side effects and consequences. Comprehensive obesity treatment programs that include medication as part of a multidisciplinary approach to weight loss and improved health outcomes must include close medical supervision and routine follow-up.

CONTRAINDICATIONS

Contraindications are situations or states in which it is not advised to use a specific drug because of the likelihood of side effects or potential risks that exceed the benefits. There are a number of medical disorders that preclude the use of Itravil (Clobenzorex), as well as specific groups for which the medication may provide serious dangers. Healthcare professionals must be aware of these contraindications in order to guarantee safe prescribing procedures and reduce patient risk. Let's examine each of these exceptions in more detail;

Heart-related Conditions:

People with a history of cardiovascular disease, such as coronary artery disease, myocardial infarction (heart attack), arrhythmias, heart failure, and stroke, should not take Itavil. Itravil's sympathomimetic effects, which can raise blood pressure, heart rate, and cardiac output, can aggravate pre-existing cardiovascular diseases and hasten cardiovascular events. Furthermore, because Itravil may have negative cardiovascular consequences, people with major cardiovascular risk factors or structural heart defects should not use this medication.

High blood pressure:

Itravil should not be used in cases of uncontrolled hypertension since it may cause blood pressure to climb even higher and raise the risk of hypertensive crises or cardiovascular events. If sympathomimetic drugs like Itravil are taken by someone with poorly controlled hypertension, they may be more vulnerable to stroke, myocardial infarction, and other consequences. As a result, blood pressure needs to be properly managed before starting Itravil therapy, and careful observation is required to guarantee that blood pressure stays within safe ranges while on medication.

Overactive Thyroid Function:

Itravil should not be used in patients with hyperthyroidism, or overactivity of the thyroid gland, as there is a risk of worsening thyroid-related symptoms and metabolic side effects. Medications known to boost thyroid hormone release and raise metabolic rate, such as Itravil, is known as a sympathomimetic. This can exacerbate symptoms of hyperthyroidism, including palpitations, tachycardia, weight loss, and heat intolerance. As a result, those who have hyperthyroidism should refrain from using Itravil and think about using other weight-loss techniques instead.

Glaucoma:

Patients with glaucoma, a disorder marked by elevated intraocular pressure and damage to the visual nerve, should not take Itravil. Medications that sympathomimetics, such as Itravil, stimulate the release of aqueous fluid and hinder it from draining from the eye, which can increase intraocular pressure. This may result in an increase in intraocular pressure and a worsening of the symptoms of glaucoma, such as optic nerve injury and vision loss. As a result, those who have glaucoma should refrain from using Itravil and instead focus on other weight-loss techniques.

Pregnancy and Nursing:

Because there could be dangers to the fetus or newborn, it is not recommended for pregnant or nursing women to take Itravil. Itravil's safety during pregnancy is unknown, and it may pass through the placenta and be eliminated in breast milk, which could expose the unborn child or growing fetus to the drug's pharmacological effects. Therefore, it is recommended that women who are pregnant or nursing refrain from using Itravil and that they think about other weight loss options.

Substance Abuse:

Itravil use should be avoided by people with a history of substance abuse, particularly abuse of stimulants, illicit drugs, or sympathomimetic pharmaceuticals, as there is a risk of overuse, dependency, and addiction. Because of their stimulating effects, sympathomimetic drugs like Itravil have a high potential for abuse and may be sought after by people with a history of substance abuse. Therefore, when giving Itravil to people who have a history of substance dependence, thorough monitoring and supervision are required, and other weight loss methods should be taken into account.

Extreme Agitation:

Itravil should not be used in cases of severe anxiety or agitation because of the stimulant properties of the medication, which can make these conditions worse. Itravil use should be avoided by people who already have anxiety disorders, panic disorders, or other mental illnesses marked by extreme agitation or anxiety since it may exacerbate symptoms and cause psychological distress or exacerbate underlying mental illnesses. Therefore, before starting Itravil medication, those with significant anxiety or agitation should be thoroughly evaluated, and other weight loss methods should be taken into account.

MAOIs, or monoamine oxidase Inhibitors:

Monoamine oxidase inhibitors (MAOIs) and Itravil should not be used together because of the possibility of potentially fatal interactions such as hypertensive crises, serotonin syndrome, and extreme stimulation of the central nervous system. Norepinephrine, dopamine, and serotonin are among the neurotransmitters whose metabolism is inhibited by MAOIs, but their release is increased and their reuptake is inhibited by sympathomimetic drugs like Itravil. As a result, using Itravil and MAOIs at the same time may cause an excessive buildup of neurotransmitters as well as other side effects.

Before beginning Itravil medication, people taking MAOIs should stop using them. It is also usually advised to wait at least 14 days for the body to clear up MAOIs before beginning Itravil treatment.

In summary, anyone with a history of substance misuse, severe anxiety or agitation, glaucoma, uncontrolled hypertension, hyperthyroidism, cardiovascular illness, breastfeeding, glaucoma, and concurrent MAOI usage should not take Itravil. These contraindications highlight the need for cautious patient selection and close medical monitoring when administering Itravil and highlight the possible dangers connected to its usage in these populations. Before starting Itravil treatment, healthcare professionals should carefully assess patients for contraindications. If a patient is not a good candidate for pharmaceutical therapy, they should also take other weight-loss methods into consideration. To guarantee the safe and efficient use of Itravil in the treatment of obesity and related disorders, frequent monitoring and follow-up are crucial.

PRECAUTIONS AND WARNINGS

In order to reduce the possibility of side effects and guarantee the safe and efficient use of the medicine, healthcare professionals and patients must take into account the precautions and warnings related to the use of Itravil (Clobenzorex). These cautions and warnings cover a range of medical disorders, drug interactions, and particular populations that may require dose modifications or additional monitoring. It's essential to comprehend these safety measures and alerts in order to maximize therapeutic results and advance patient wellbeing. Let's investigate them thoroughly:

Effects on the Heart:

Because of its sympathomimetic qualities, Itravil may have cardiovascular effects such as raised blood pressure, arrhythmias, and accelerated heart rate. Consequently, people who already have high blood pressure, cardiovascular disease, or other cardiovascular risk factors should use caution while administering Itravil. Throughout Itravil treatment, it is imperative to closely monitor vital indicators such as blood pressure and heart rate in order to spot any changes that could indicate cardiovascular side effects. Furthermore, before starting Itravil therapy, those with a history of cardiovascular events should be thoroughly assessed; in this population, other weight-loss methods may need to be taken into account.

Psychological Impacts:

Itravil and other sympathomimetic drugs may make mental health issues worse. These illnesses include bipolar disorder, anxiety, agitation, and psychosis. As a result, care should be used while giving Itravil to people who have a history of mental illness or mood disorders. Throughout Itravil medication, patients must be closely observed for any changes in mood, behavior, or mental state. They should also be instructed to report any new or worsening psychiatric symptoms to their healthcare professional. When using Itravil, those with a history of mental illnesses may need closer supervision and assistance; if psychiatric symptoms develop, other options for weight loss should be explored.

Risk of Seizures:

Itravil and other sympathomimetic drugs have been linked to a higher risk of seizures, especially in people with epilepsy or a history of seizures. Itravil should therefore be used with caution in this population and caution should be used when giving it to people who have a history of seizure disorders.

It is imperative to closely monitor patients receiving Itravil for signs of seizure activity, such as altered awareness, rigidity in the muscles, or convulsions. When taking Itravil, those with a history of seizures should be constantly watched, and if they experience seizure activity, they should think about other weight-loss options.

Potential for Substance Abuse:

Particularly in those with a history of substance abuse or addiction, sympathomimetic drugs such as Itravil carry the risk of misuse, dependence, and addiction. Itravil should therefore be used with caution in this demographic and caution should be used when prescribing it to people who have a history of substance dependence. Throughout Itravil treatment, careful observation is required for indications of abuse, dependence, or addiction, such as drug-seeking behavior, tolerance, and withdrawal symptoms. When taking Itravil, people with a history of substance abuse should be constantly watched, and if overuse or dependence are noticed, other weight-loss methods may need to be explored.

Impairment of Renal Function:

Renal impairment, especially in those with end-stage renal disease or severe renal impairment, may impact the pharmacokinetics of Itravil and raise the risk of negative consequences. Itravil should therefore be used with caution in this population and caution should be used when administering it to anyone with renal impairment. Continual monitoring for side effects is necessary throughout Itravil treatment, and dose modifications may be required depending on the severity of renal impairment. When taking Itravil, people with severe renal impairment should be continuously watched, and if side effects arise, other weight-loss options may be taken into consideration.

Hepatic Deficit:

Hepatic impairment, especially in those with severe liver disease or impairment, may impact the pharmacokinetics of Itravil and raise the possibility of side events. Itravil should therefore be used with caution in this population and caution should be used when prescribing it to people with hepatic impairment. The degree of hepatic impairment may require dose modifications, and careful observation for side effects is required when using Itravil. When taking Itravil, people with severe hepatic impairment should be continuously watched, and if side effects arise, other options for weight loss may be taken into consideration.

Itravil side effects, cardiovascular effects, psychiatric side effects, seizure risk, medication interactions, potential for substance misuse, renal impairment, hepatic impairment, elderly population, pregnancy, and breastfeeding are all included in the list of cautions and warnings related to its use. Before starting Itravil treatment, healthcare professionals should thoroughly assess each patient for these risks. For those who are more likely to experience side effects, they should also take other weight-loss methods into consideration. Itravil must be used carefully and with a customized treatment plan in order to be used safely in the treatment of obesity and associated disorders.

ADVERSE REACTIONS

Itravil (Clobenzorex) adverse responses include a broad spectrum of possible side effects that could manifest while undergoing treatment. The degree of these adverse responses can vary, and they may impact many organ systems, such as the neurological, gastrointestinal, metabolic, mental, and cardiovascular systems. It is essential for patients and healthcare professionals to be aware of the possible side effects of Itravil in order to identify and appropriately handle these consequences. Let's examine these negative effects in more detail;

Adverse Cardiovascular Reactions:

Some of the most frequent and alarming adverse effects of using Itravil are reactions that impact the cardiovascular system. These could consist of;

- Tachycardia: The stimulatory effects of sympathomimetic drugs, such as Itravil, frequently cause an increase in heart rate as a side effect.
- Hypertension: Increased sympathetic activity and peripheral vasoconstriction brought on by Itravil may result in elevated blood pressure.
- Arrhythmias: The drug's effects on cardiac conduction pathways may result in

arrhythmias, such as palpitations, atrial fibrillation, and ventricular arrhythmias.

- Myocardial Ischemia: This condition, which is more common in those with underlying coronary artery disease, is characterized by decreased coronary blood flow and an imbalance in the oxygen supply-demand in the heart. It can result in angina or myocardial infarction.

- Cardiovascular Events: Using sympathomimetic drugs like Itravil has been linked to serious cardiovascular events, such as stroke, heart attack, and sudden cardiac death. This relationship is especially evident in people who already have cardiovascular disease. During Itravil treatment, medical professionals should keep an eye out for symptoms of cardiovascular adverse reactions in patients, such as changes in heart rate, blood pressure, and cardiac rhythm. Individuals who have a history of cardiovascular disease or who already have cardiovascular risk factors may need to be closely monitored and may need to explore other weight loss options.

Adverse Reactions to the Central Nervous System:

Itravil side effects that impact the central nervous system are also frequent and can includes;

- Insomnia: Itravil's stimulatory effects on the central nervous system may make it difficult to fall asleep or stay asleep.
- Headache: Commonly seen as a side effect of sympathomimetic drugs such as Itravil, headaches can be linked to changes in neurotransmitter levels or increased cerebral blood flow.
- Dizziness: Variations in blood pressure or brain perfusion can cause feelings of lightheadedness or vertigo, especially when standing up fast.
- Nervousness: The drug's stimulatory effects on the central nervous system may lead to increased anxiety, restlessness, or agitation.
- Tremor: Excessive sympathetic activity and neuromuscular excitability can result in fine tremors or shaking of the hands or other extremities.
- Seizures: Despite being uncommon, seizures have been linked to the use of sympathomimetic drugs like Itravil, especially in people with a history of epilepsy or seizures.

It is recommended that patients notify their healthcare practitioner of any adverse reactions involving the central nervous system. In the event that these symptoms become unpleasant or persistent, Itravil dosage modifications or withdrawal may be indicated.

Reactions Adverse to the Gastrointestinal:

Itravil therapy may result in gastrointestinal adverse events, which could include the following:
- Dry Mouth: The anticholinergic effects of the medication may result in decreased salivation and dry mouth.
- Constipation: Difficulty passing stools or constipation may result from decreased gastrointestinal motility and transit time.
- Nausea or Vomiting: During the first several weeks of Itravil treatment, nausea and vomiting are common side effects of digestive disturbance.
- Abdominal Discomfort: Changes in visceral feeling or gastrointestinal motility may result in dyspepsia, abdominal pain, or discomfort.
- Diarrhea: Though less frequent, changes in stool consistency or an increase in gastrointestinal motility can both lead to diarrhea.

To assist prevent gastrointestinal side events, patients should be advised to keep a nutritious diet high in fiber and to drink plenty of water. Patients should speak with their healthcare physician for additional assessment and treatment if symptoms intensify or continue.

Adverse Psychiatric Reactions:

Itravil therapy may result in adverse effects that impact mood, behavior, and cognitive function. These reactions can include;

- Anxiety or Agitation: People who are prone to anxiety or psychiatric illnesses may experience increased anxiety, restlessness, or agitation.
- Increased central nervous system arousal or stimulation may be the cause of insomnia or sleep disturbances, which are characterized by difficulty falling or staying asleep.
- Mood swings or irritability: Modifications in neurotransmitter levels or central nervous system activity can lead to mood swings, emotional lability, or irritation.
- Psychosis or Hallucinations: The use of sympathomimetic drugs such as Itravil has been linked, however infrequently, to psychotic symptoms such as hallucinations, delusions, or paranoia.

It is recommended that patients notify their healthcare practitioner of any alterations in their mood or behavior. In the event of psychiatric adverse effects, Itravil dosage modifications or withdrawal may be required.

Adverse Metabolic Reactions:

During Itravil medication, the following adverse effects may occur that impact metabolism and endocrine function;

- Weight Loss: Although losing weight is the intended therapeutic outcome of Itravil, people who already suffer from malnutrition or eating disorders may have excessive or quick weight loss.
- Blood glucose levels can fluctuate due to variations in insulin sensitivity and glucose metabolism. This is especially true for those with diabetes or impaired glucose tolerance.
- Electrolyte Imbalance: Elevated metabolic rate and electrolyte excretion in the urine can lead to changes in fluid and electrolyte balance, including hypokalemia and hyponatremia.

During Itravil treatment, healthcare professionals should keep an eye out for changes in a patient's weight, blood sugar, and electrolyte balance, especially if the patient has a history of metabolic disorders or other risk factors.

Additional Adverse Outcomes:

Additional negative effects associated with Itravil use include;

- Allergic Reactions: The usage of sympathomimetic drugs like Itravil has been linked to hypersensitivity reactions, which include rash, itching, urticaria, angioedema, and anaphylaxis.

- Ocular Effects: People who are prone to ocular diseases may experience blurred vision, mydriasis (dilation of the pupil), and other visual disturbances.
- Urinary Retention: The anticholinergic effects of the medication on the bladder may cause difficulty urinating or urine retention.

In conclusion, there are a variety of possible side effects that could have an impact on different organ systems that are included in the adverse reactions linked to Itravil use. During Itravil treatment, healthcare professionals should regularly monitor patients for indications of adverse reactions and modify therapy as necessary to reduce the risk of problems. Patients should be informed about the possible side effects of Itravil and urged to notify their healthcare provider right away if they experience any new or unusual symptoms. Optimizing treatment outcomes and promoting patient safety when using Itravil requires close monitoring, tailored treatment plans, and open communication between patients and healthcare professionals.

DRUG INTERACTIONS

When using drugs like Itravil (Clobenzorex) safely and effectively, drug interactions are a crucial factor to take into account. When two or more medications are used together, there may be interactions that change the pharmacokinetic or pharmacodynamic characteristics of the drugs and may result in side effects or decreased efficacy. Healthcare professionals must be aware of possible drug interactions in order to prevent negative consequences and improve patient care. Let's examine Itravil medication interactions in more detail;

Serotonin-Norepinephrine Reuptake Inhibitors (SNRIs) and Selective Serotonin Reuptake Inhibitors (SSRIs):

The risk of serotonin syndrome, a potentially fatal illness marked by symptoms like agitation, confusion, hallucinations, hyperthermia, diaphoresis, tremor, and autonomic instability, may rise if Itravil is used concurrently with SSRIs or SNRIs. Serotonin levels in the brain are raised by both Itravil and SSRIs/SNRIs; taking these drugs together may result in excessive serotonin buildup and toxicity. As a result, care should be taken while giving Itravil alongside SSRIs or SNRIs, and patients should be continuously watched for serotonin syndrome symptoms.

TCAs, or tricyclic Antidepressants:

Because Itravil and TCAs have additive sympathomimetic effects, taking them together may raise the risk of cardiovascular side effects such as tachycardia, hypertension, and arrhythmias. While sympathomimetic drugs like Itravil increase the release and decrease the reuptake of norepinephrine and serotonin, TCAs block their reuptake, increasing the amount of these neurotransmitters in the synaptic cleft. As a result, using Itravil and TCAs at the same time may cause adverse cardiovascular consequences and excessive sympathetic activation. When providing Itravil concurrently with TCAs, healthcare practitioners should regularly monitor patients for evidence of cardiovascular effects. Dosage modifications may be required to limit the risk of adverse responses.

Sympathomimetic Drugs:

Because of the additive sympathomimetic effects of Itravil, concurrent use with other sympathomimetic medications, such as decongestants, appetite suppressants, or stimulants, may raise the risk of cardiovascular side effects, such as tachycardia, hypertension, and arrhythmias. Combining sympathomimetic drugs can cause cardiovascular toxicity and excessive sympathetic activation, especially in people who already have cardiovascular illness or risk factors. Consequently, care should be used while giving Itravil together with other sympathomimetic medications, and patients should be continuously watched for any indications of cardiovascular side effects.

Low Blood Pressure Drugs:

The antihypertensive effects of beta-blockers, calcium channel blockers, and angiotensin-converting enzyme (ACE) inhibitors may be counteracted and the risk of hypertension increased when Itravil is taken concurrently with these drugs. Antihypertensive drugs, which try to lower blood pressure, can be counteracted by sympathomimetic medications, such as Itravil, which can raise blood pressure and heart rate. Consequently, while prescribing Itravil together with antihypertensive drugs, careful blood pressure monitoring is required, and dose modifications can be required to keep blood pressure within goal ranges.

Antidiabetic Medicines:

When Itravil and antidiabetic drugs like insulin or oral hypoglycemic medicines are used together, blood glucose levels may change and the dosage of the antidiabetic drug may need to be adjusted. Blood glucose levels may fluctuate as a result of sympathomimetic drugs such as Itravil, which can worsen glucose tolerance and raise insulin resistance. As a result, when giving Itravil together with antidiabetic drugs, careful monitoring of blood glucose levels is required, and dose modifications can be required to maintain glycemic control.

Anticoagulants Other Than Warfarin:

When warfarin or other anticoagulants are taken concurrently with Itravil, the effects of these drugs may change and the risk of bleeding may rise. Medications designed to stimulate the heart, such as Itravil, can raise blood pressure and heart rate. This can result in an increase in cardiac output and possible changes to blood coagulation. Therefore, when administering Itravil concurrently with warfarin or other anticoagulants, close monitoring of prothrombin time (PT) or international normalized ratio (INR) is required, and dose modifications may be required to maintain therapeutic anticoagulation.

Antipsychotics and Antidepressants:

Because of the additive pharmacodynamic effects, using Itravil concurrently with antidepressants or antipsychotics may raise the risk of cardiovascular side effects, serotonin syndrome, or other severe reactions. Medications known to stimulate neurotransmitter levels in the brain, such as Itravil, can cause changes in mood, behavior, and heart rate. Consequently, care should be taken when giving Itravil along with antidepressants or antipsychotics, and patients should be continuously watched for any indications of a negative reaction.

CYP2D6 Inducers and Inhibitors:

The primary metabolite of Itravil is CYP2D6, a cytochrome P450 enzyme. As a result, using CYP2D6 inducers or inhibitors along with Itravil may change the drug's pharmacokinetic characteristics and metabolism. Itravil plasma concentrations may rise in response to CYP2D6 inhibitors such fluoxetine, paroxetine, and quinidine. This could improve pharmacodynamic effects and raise the possibility of negative responses. On the other hand, CYP2D6 inducers including phenytoin, carbamazepine, and rifampin may lower Itravil plasma concentrations, decreasing its effectiveness and possibly resulting in treatment failure. Consequently, care should be used while administering Itravil along with CYP2D6 inducers or inhibitors, and dose modifications might be required to maximize therapy.

In conclusion, pharmacokinetic and pharmacodynamic aspects of many drugs may be affected by drug interactions with Itravil, which may result in unfavorable consequences or decreased efficacy. Prior to starting Itravil treatment, medical professionals should thoroughly evaluate patients' prescription schedules and take into account any possible drug interactions. To effectively identify and manage drug interactions, patients must be closely monitored. To maximize therapy and reduce the risk of unfavorable outcomes, dose modifications or other treatment approaches may be required. In order to reduce the possibility of drug interactions, patients should be informed about the possible side effects of Itravil and encouraged to disclose to their healthcare practitioner all of the medications they use, including prescription, over-the-counter, and dietary supplements.

OVERDOSE

Because of Itravil's (Clobenzorex) sympathomimetic qualities and central nervous system stimulant effects, overdosing on the medication can have major, potentially fatal consequences. An overdose happens when a person takes more medication than is advised or prescribed, which leaves the body with toxic amounts of the substance. For medical professionals to treat patients who have overdosed on Itravil promptly and appropriately, they must have a thorough understanding of the signs, symptoms, and management of this condition. Let's examine Itravil overdose in more detail:

Clinical Display:

Depending on the amount consumed, the person's tolerance to sympathomimetic drugs, and the existence of underlying medical conditions, the clinical appearance of an Itravil overdose can change. Itravil overdose symptoms and indicators frequently includes;

- Cardiovascular Effects: The drug's sympathomimetic effects on the cardiovascular system may result in tachycardia (fast heart rate), hypertension (high blood pressure), palpitations, arrhythmias (irregular heart beats), and chest pain.

- Central Nervous System Effects: The stimulatory effects of the medication on the central nervous system may include agitation, restlessness, anxiety, disorientation, hallucinations, delirium, tremors, seizures, and coma.
- Gastrointestinal Effects: Changes in visceral feeling and gastrointestinal motility may result in nausea, vomiting, abdominal discomfort, and diarrhea.
- Effects on the Respiratory System: Enhanced sympathetic activity and higher metabolic demand may lead to tachypnea, or fast breathing, and respiratory distress.
- Metabolic Effects: Increased metabolic rate and catecholamine release may lead to hyperthermia (high body temperature), metabolic acidosis, and rhabdomyolysis (muscle breakdown).

Supervisory:

Supportive care, disinfection, laboratory parameter and vital sign monitoring, and symptomatic treatment of sequelae are all part of managing an Itravil overdose. Important managerial facets could be;

- Decontamination: If the overdose happens within a few hours after intake and the patient is compliant and attentive, consider stomach lavage or the injection of activated charcoal to limit absorption of the medication. However, because of the potential for consequences, gastric lavage is generally not advised in individuals who are asymptomatic or only mildly symptomatic.
- Symptomatic Management: Attend to issues and symptoms as they emerge. Give benzodiazepines to treat anxiety, seizures, or agitation. For hypertension and tachycardia, use beta-blockers or calcium channel blockers. In order to treat hyperthermia, give antipyretics and supportive care. Keep an eye on the acid-base balance and electrolyte levels, and adjust any irregularities as necessary.
- Enhanced Elimination: In extreme cases or when supporting measures are not working, think about hemodialysis or hemoperfusion. Nevertheless, these therapies are not very

effective at getting rid of sympathomimetic medications like Itravil.

Observing:

Keep a watchful eye on the patient's vital signs, mental state, heart health, and electrolyte balance. Conduct ECGs in succession to check for myocardial ischemia and arrhythmias. Assess metabolic and respiratory status by measuring arterial blood gases (ABGs), serum electrolytes, and creatinine kinase (CK). If the situation is severe, think about being admitted to an intensive care unit (ICU) for close observation and treatment.

Problems:

Cardiovascular collapse, myocardial infarction, stroke, rhabdomyolysis, renal failure, metabolic acidosis, respiratory failure, and death are among the complications that might arise from an Itravil overdose. Timely identification and management of complications is crucial in reducing overdose-related morbidity and death.

Effects Over Time:

Long-term consequences from an Itravil overdose could include cognitive impairment, mental illnesses, heart problems, and kidney problems.

Assessing and managing these possible problems may need close monitoring and follow-up.

Avoidance:

In order to prevent Itravil overdose, patients must be informed about the dangers of overdosing, abuse, and incorrect dosage as well as how to take the medicine. When it is acceptable, healthcare professionals should take into account alternate treatment approaches in addition to closely evaluating individuals for risk factors for overdose, such as a history of substance misuse, mental health issues, and cardiovascular illness.

To sum up, the sympathomimetic and central nervous system stimulant actions of Itravil can lead to severe and potentially fatal consequences in the event of an overdose. Effective handling of overdose situations requires prompt recognition, supportive care, and symptomatic therapy. To limit morbidity and mortality associated with overdose, healthcare personnel should possess knowledge of the clinical presentation, management guidelines, and probable sequelae of Itravil overdose.

SPECIAL POPULATIONS

The term "special populations" describes sets of people who may have particular traits, circumstances, or other factors that may have an impact on the safety, effectiveness, pharmacokinetics, or pharmacodynamics of drugs like Itravil (Clobenzorex). Pediatric patients, elderly patients, women in pregnancy, nursing moms, people with hepatic or renal impairment, and people with comorbid conditions including mental illness, substance misuse disorders, or cardiovascular disease are some examples of these populations. Healthcare professionals must comprehend the particular requirements and concerns of these distinct populations in order to maximize treatment results and guarantee patient safety. Let's take a closer look at the unique populations connected to Itravil use;

Young Patients:

There is a dearth of information on Itravil's effectiveness and safety in young patients. It is generally not advised for children and teenagers to utilize sympathomimetic drugs, such as Itravil, for weight loss because of possible negative effects on growth, development, and cardiovascular health. The cardiovascular and central nervous system side effects of sympathomimetic medications, such as tachycardia, hypertension, sleeplessness, and agitation, may be more common in pediatric patients. As such, alternate methods of weight loss should be taken into account for juvenile patients, and Itravil use in this population should be handled carefully.

Elderly Individuals:

The pharmacokinetics, pharmacodynamics, and organ function of sympathomimetic drugs, such as Itravil, may alter with age, making elderly patients more vulnerable to its side effects. When taking Itravil, elderly people may be more susceptible to cardiovascular events, psychological side effects, and stimulation of their central nervous system. Consequently, care should be used while providing Itravil to elderly individuals, as they may benefit from lower starting doses. It's important to closely monitor any negative effects, and in the event that they do arise, alternate weight loss plans should be taken into account.

Expectant Mothers:

Because there could be dangers to the fetus, it is not recommended for pregnant women to use Itravil. Medication that sympathomimetics, such as Itravil, can enter the placenta and impact fetal development, resulting in unfavorable consequences like stunted growth, premature birth, and withdrawal symptoms in the newborn. When a pregnant woman finds out she is pregnant, she should be urged to stop taking Itravil right away and think about other weight-loss options. Healthcare professionals should give adequate prenatal care and keep a close eye on pregnant patients who have been exposed to Itravil for any potential negative effects on fetal development.

Nursing Mother:

Itravil should not be administered to nursing women because of possible dangers to the unborn child. Medications known to cause sympathomimetic effects, such as Itravil, might impact breastfeeding infants and cause side effects including agitation, poor eating, and weight loss. These drugs can also enter breast milk. It is advisable to counsel nursing mothers to stop using Itravil and think about alternate breastfeeding-friendly weight-loss techniques. In order to support breastfeeding and the health of the unborn child, medical professionals should advise nursing moms on the significance of sustaining a healthy diet and level of hydration when stopping Itravil.

Hepatic Deficit:

Itravil's metabolism and clearance can be impacted by hepatic impairment, which may change the drug's pharmacokinetics and raise the risk of side effects. Hepatic impairment patients may need to start with lower doses of Itravil and be closely watched for any signs of toxicity. When treating patients with hepatic impairment with Itravil, close monitoring of liver function tests is required, and dose modifications may be required depending on the severity of hepatic dysfunction. When it comes to people with significant liver impairment, alternative weight loss methods should be taken into account.

Impairment of Renal Function:

Renal impairment may modify the pharmacokinetics and may raise the risk of side effects by affecting the excretion and clearance of drugs such as Itravil. People who have impaired kidney function might need to start with lower doses of Itravil and be closely watched for any hazardous symptoms. Patients with renal impairment must have close monitoring of their electrolytes and renal function while receiving Itravil; depending on the severity of their renal impairment, dose modifications may also be required. Patients with severe renal impairment should be evaluated for other weight loss options.

Heart-related Conditions:

Those who take sympathomimetic drugs, such as Itravil, may be more vulnerable to adverse cardiovascular events if they already have cardiovascular disease. These people might be more prone to myocardial ischemia, hypertension, arrhythmias, and tachycardia. As a result, patients with cardiovascular illness should use caution when prescribed Itravil, and careful monitoring of vital signs and heart function is required throughout treatment. Patients with substantial cardiovascular risk factors should think about other weight loss methods.

Psychiatric Conditions:

People who suffer from mental health conditions like anxiety, depression, bipolar disorder, or psychosis could be particularly vulnerable to the psychological side effects of drugs that stimulate the sympathetic nervous system, such as Itravil. When using Itravil, these people may develop an increase in psychiatric symptoms such as agitation, anxiety, sleeplessness, or psychosis. Consequently, patients with psychiatric illnesses should be prescribed Itravil with caution, and treatment requires close monitoring of mental status and mood. Those with substantial psychiatric comorbidity should think about other weight loss techniques.

Drug Abuse Disorders:

People who have previously struggled with substance abuse or addiction may be more susceptible to misusing, abusing, or becoming dependent on sympathomimetic drugs such as Itravil. When using Itravil, these people may be more likely to experience tolerance, withdrawal symptoms, or obsessive drug-seeking behavior. As a result, individuals with drug abuse disorders should be prescribed Itravil with caution, and during therapy, careful observation for indications of abuse or dependency is required. For those who have a history of substance abuse or addiction, alternative weight loss techniques should be taken into consideration.

In conclusion, pediatric and geriatric patients, women who are pregnant or nursing, people with hepatic or renal impairment, and people who have comorbid conditions like cardiovascular disease, mental health issues, or substance abuse disorders are among the special populations that need to be taken into account when prescribing Itravil. Healthcare professionals should carefully evaluate any risks associated with these groups and modify treatment regimens as necessary to maximize safety and effectiveness while lowering the possibility of side effects. The safe and efficient use of Itravil in specific populations requires close observation and tailored treatment.

CLINICAL STUDIES

To assess the safety, effectiveness, and tolerability of drugs such as Itravil (Clobenzorex) in different patient populations, clinical studies are crucial. Strict scientific procedures and ethical concerns are used in these research to produce trustworthy data that guides regulatory approval procedures and healthcare decision-making. Preclinical research, Phase I trials for safety evaluation, Phase II trials for preliminary efficacy evaluation, Phase III trials for confirmatory efficacy and safety assessment, and Phase IV trials for post-marketing surveillance are the typical clinical studies of Itravil. Let's take a closer look at the Itravil clinical trials that were carried out;

Preclinical Investigations:

Prior to a medicine being tested on humans, preclinical research is carried out in lab settings and on animals. Preclinical research on Itravil may involve toxicological evaluations, pharmacokinetic studies, mechanism of action analyses, and pharmacological profiling. Insights about the drug's pharmacological characteristics, safety profile, and possible therapeutic pathways are gained from these research, which help with study design and dosage selection for upcoming clinical trials.

Clinical Trials in Phase I:

The initial phase of human testing, known as phase I clinical trials, is devoted to evaluating a drug's safety, tolerability, pharmacokinetics, and pharmacodynamics in healthy volunteers or those who have the intended ailment. The goal of Itravil's phase I studies is to detect dose-limiting toxicities, find the maximum tolerated dose, and define the drug's features related to absorption, distribution, metabolism, and excretion. These investigations offer vital information about the safety profile and preliminary pharmacological effects of Itravil in humans, which helps with the selection of doses for subsequent clinical research.

Clinical Trials in Phase II:

Phase II clinical studies are designed to assess a drug's initial efficacy and the best way to dose patients with the intended disease. In phase II trials, a larger cohort of obese or overweight individuals are usually given Itravil, and the medication's benefits are evaluated on weight loss, metabolic parameters, and safety outcomes during a predetermined treatment duration. These investigations serve to improve dosage schedules for upcoming Phase III trials and offer early proof of Itravil's therapeutic potential.

Clinical Trials in Phase III:

Large-scale, randomized, controlled investigations called phase III clinical trials are made to verify a drug's safety and effectiveness in a larger group of patients. Phase III trials of Itravil evaluate the medication's effects on weight loss, maintenance of weight loss, improvement in metabolic parameters, and long-term safety outcomes over an extended treatment period in a diverse group of obese or overweight patients compared to placebo or standard treatment. The efficacy and safety profile of Itravil are strongly supported by these trials, hence facilitating regulatory approval and clinical use.

Clinical Trials in Phase IV:

Following a medication's approval for marketing, phase IV clinical trials also referred to as post-marketing surveillance studies are carried out to track the drug's safety and efficacy in actual clinical settings. Phase IV trials for Itravil entail gathering information on side effects, long-term results, and patient adherence over an extended length of time in a larger patient group. These studies offer insightful information about the long-term safety profile and practical efficacy of Itravil, assisting in the detection of uncommon or postponed side effects and maximizing its application in therapeutic settings.

Comparative Effectiveness Study:

Comparative effectiveness research (CER) compares, in actual clinical situations, the efficacy of several treatment choices for a given ailment. In a variety of patient demographics, CER studies on Itravil may evaluate its cost-effectiveness, safety, and effectiveness against other weight-loss drugs, lifestyle changes, or bariatric surgery. Based on the relative advantages and disadvantages of Itravil in comparison to other interventions, these studies offer useful information that patients and healthcare professionals can use to make well-informed treatment decisions.

Pharmacogenomics and Subgroup Analysis:

Clinical trials may incorporate subgroup analyses and pharmacogenomic studies to assess the efficacy of Itravil in particular patient subpopulations or individuals with genetic variations that impact drug response. Subgroup analyses offer valuable information about the potential variability in clinical outcomes of Itravil by evaluating its efficacy and safety across various age groups, genders, ethnicities, and comorbidity profiles. Pharmacogenomic research may reveal genetic markers linked to a variable Itravil response or susceptibility to side effects, allowing for individualized treatment plans based on unique genetic profiles.

Long-Term Follow-Up Studies:

To assess Itravil's continued safety, effectiveness, and tolerability across longer treatment periods than the original clinical trials, long-term follow-up studies may be carried out. In patients undergoing long-term Itravil medication, these studies may evaluate the maintenance of weight loss, metabolic results, cardiovascular events, and long-term adverse effects. In real-world clinical practice, long-term follow-up data offer important insights on the longevity of Itravil's effects and how it affects overall health outcomes.

To sum up, Itravil clinical studies cover a wide range of research activities, including preclinical studies, Phase I–IV trials, and postmarketing surveillance. In order to support clinical decision-making and enhance patient care, these studies offer crucial information on the safety, effectiveness, and practical usefulness of Itravil in a variety of patient categories. In order to safely and effectively integrate Itravil into clinical practice for the management of obesity and related diseases, more study is required to clarify the therapeutic potential and long-term effects associated with its use.

REGULATORY STATUS

The approval, labeling, and monitoring of a drug such as Itravil (Clobenzorex) by regulatory bodies tasked with guaranteeing the efficacy, safety, and caliber of pharmaceuticals are referred to as its regulatory status. Obtaining regulatory approval entails a stringent assessment procedure that assesses the preclinical and clinical evidence bolstering the drug's benefit-risk profile and conformity to regulatory requirements. Let's take a closer look at Itravil's regulatory situation:

Regulatory Organizations:

Governmental organizations in charge of drug regulation and oversight normally approve pharmaceuticals. Depending on the nation or area in which Itravil is sold, several regulatory bodies may be involved in the approval process. Pharmaceutical products are governed by the Food and medication Administration (FDA) in the United States, and medication regulation in the European Union is managed by the European Medicines Agency (EMA). Similar functions may be assigned to national regulatory bodies in other nations.
Submission of Regulations:

Upon completion of clinical trials and gathering enough data to substantiate Itravil's safety and effectiveness, the pharmaceutical company files a New Drug Application (NDA) or Marketing Authorization Application (MAA) for regulatory agency evaluation. Comprehensive information on the drug's pharmacology, pharmacokinetics, clinical efficacy, safety profile, manufacturing procedures, and labeling is included in the application.

- Regulatory Review: To evaluate Itravil's benefit-risk profile and decide if it satisfies the requirements for approval, regulatory bodies carefully examine the evidence that has been presented. The evaluation procedure assesses the suitability of the suggested risk management and labeling techniques in addition to the accuracy, consistency, and quality of the data. To help them make decisions, regulatory reviewers may confer with advisory groups and impartial specialists.

- Labeling and prescription Information: The regulatory body gives a marketing authorization and approves the labeling and prescription information for Itravil if the drug is approved. Indications, dosage and administration guidelines, contraindications, cautions and warnings, adverse reactions, drug interactions, and usage in particular populations (e.g., pediatric, geriatric, pregnant, or nursing patients) are just a few of the critical details that are provided on labels to patients and healthcare professionals.

- Post-Marketing Surveillance: Following approval, regulatory bodies use post-marketing surveillance programs to keep an eye on Itravil's efficacy and safety. These applications gather and examine information on side effects, prescription mistakes, and additional safety issues related to the usage of Itravil in actual clinical settings. To address found safety risks, regulatory bodies may mandate that the drug sponsor carry out post-marketing research or put risk management plans into place.

- Updates to the Regulatory Status: If new safety or efficacious information becomes available after approval, regulatory bodies may decide to revise the regulatory status of Itravil. This could entail sending out safety announcements, updating the information on the label, making changes to prescription instructions, or putting new legal restrictions or regulatory requirements on the use of the medication. Periodic reviews of licensed pharmaceuticals are carried out by regulatory agencies to guarantee continued adherence to regulatory requirements.

- International Harmonization: Regulatory bodies work together globally to standardize regulations and expedite the timely licensing of drugs in various jurisdictions. In order to improve regulatory efficiency and consistency, this involves exchanging information and best practices, aligning requirements and review processes, and reciprocal acknowledgment of regulatory decisions. The goal of international harmonization efforts is to maintain high standards of safety and efficacy while streamlining the worldwide medication development and licensing process.

To summarize, Itravil's regulatory status entails a thorough assessment process carried out by regulatory bodies to assess the medication's quality, safety, and efficacy. With regulatory permission, Itravil can be prescribed and sold to treat obesity or overweight, provided that it complies with regulations and is continuously monitored after the product is sold. By ensuring that drugs like Itravil adhere to strict regulations and are used safely and effectively in clinical practice, regulatory bodies play a crucial role in protecting the public's health.

CONCLUSION

Itravil, also known as Clobenzorex, is a medication that can be used to treat obesity or overweight. This gives medical professionals a means of addressing a serious health issue that affects millions of people globally. We have examined every facet of Itravil in this thorough investigation, covering everything from its pharmacological profile and mode of action to its clinical efficacy, safety concerns, and regulatory status. Itravil works mainly through its sympathomimetic qualities, which suppress appetite, boost energy expenditure, and improve fat metabolism in order to aid in weight loss. Because of these effects, it's a useful addition to dietary therapies, behavioral therapy, and lifestyle changes in the treatment of obesity, especially for those with major comorbidities or trouble accomplishing weight loss objectives with non-pharmacological means alone.

It's important to understand that using Itravil carries some hazards, nevertheless. Adverse reactions highlight the significance of careful patient selection, monitoring, and adherence to prescribing guidelines. These reactions can include cardiovascular consequences, mental symptoms, and the potential for misuse or dependence. Due to their specialized considerations and susceptibility to negative effects, special populations, such as pediatric, geriatric, pregnant, or breastfeeding persons, as well as those with hepatic or renal impairment or comorbidities, require special attention. For Itravil to be used safely and effectively in clinical practice, post-marketing surveillance, regulatory control, and clinical trials are essential. Carefully considered research, carried out in compliance with legal and ethical guidelines, gives rise to evidence-based choices and educates medical professionals on the advantages, dangers, and best practices of a given drug.

In the end, a comprehensive strategy emphasizing patient education, customized treatment plans, close monitoring, and cooperation between healthcare providers and patients is necessary for the successful integration of Itravil into clinical practice. Healthcare providers can optimize the potential benefits of Itravil while minimizing its associated risks by utilizing existing evidence, following prescribed guidelines, and placing a high priority on patient safety and well-being. This will ultimately improve outcomes and quality of life for individuals who are grappling with obesity or being overweight.